Copyright © 2019 by Lucas B. Mark

Disclaimer

All Right Reserved. No part of this book may be reproduced or transmitted in any form or by any means, mechanical or electronic, including photocopying or reccording, or by any information storage and retrieval system, or transmitted by email without permission in writting from pubisher. The views expressed are those of the author alone.

ABC
BOOK OF FRUIT

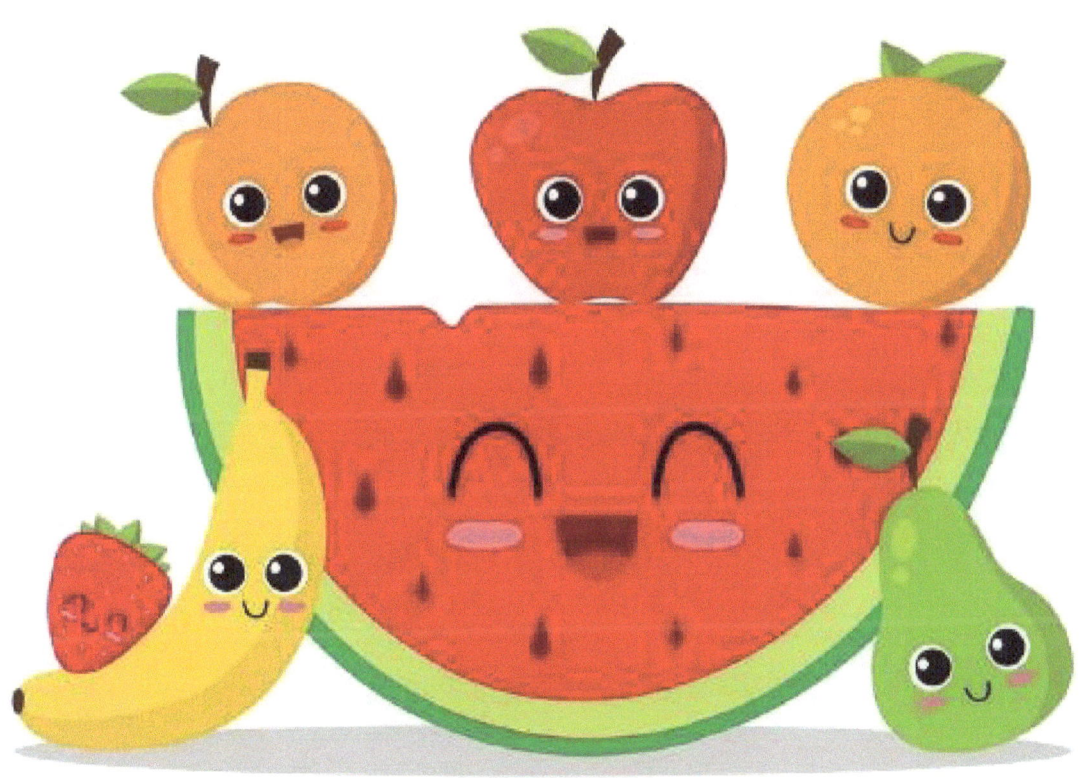

FOR KIDS WHO LOVE FRUIT
AGES 1-4

A a

is for Apple

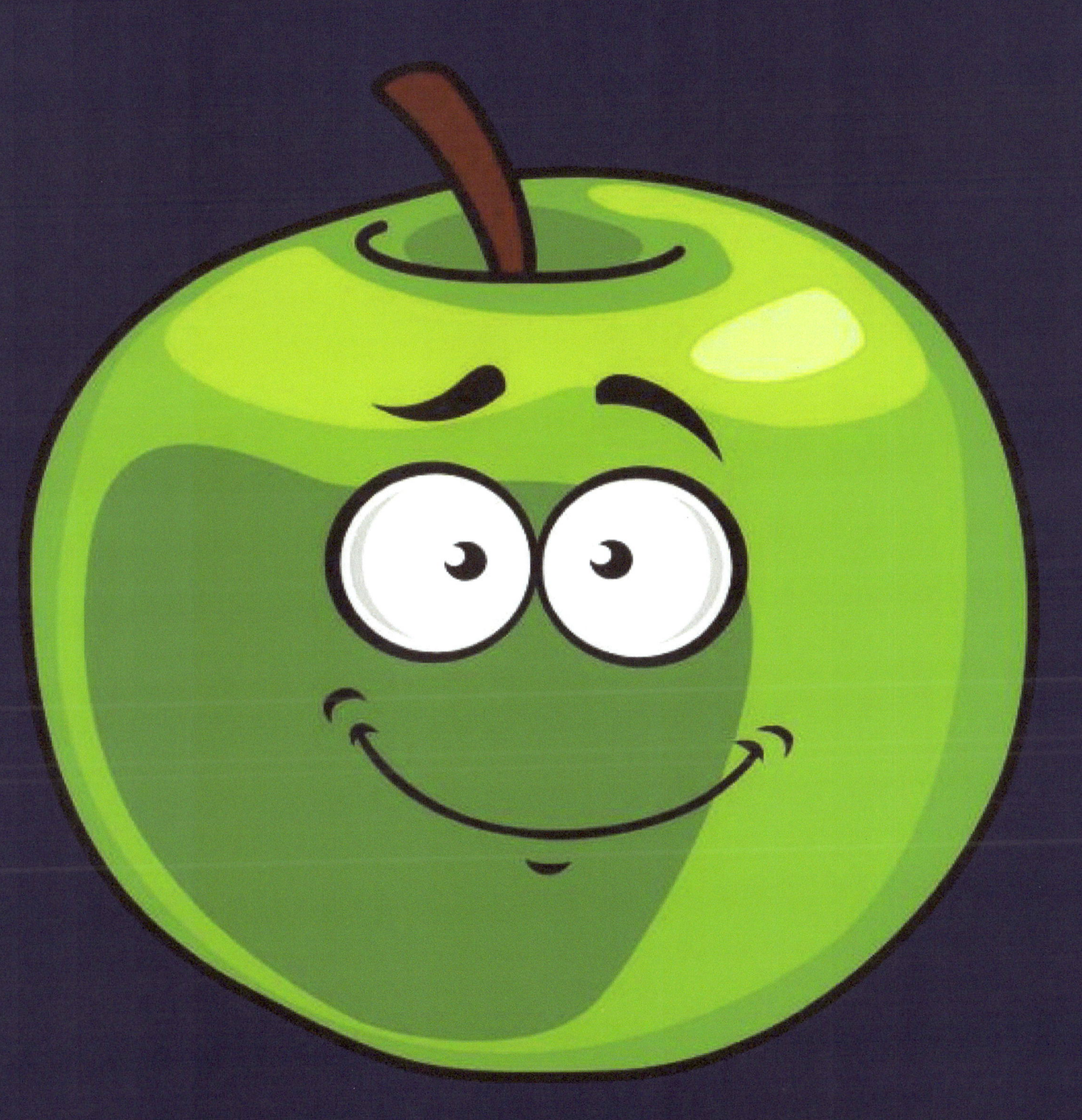

B b

is for Blueberry

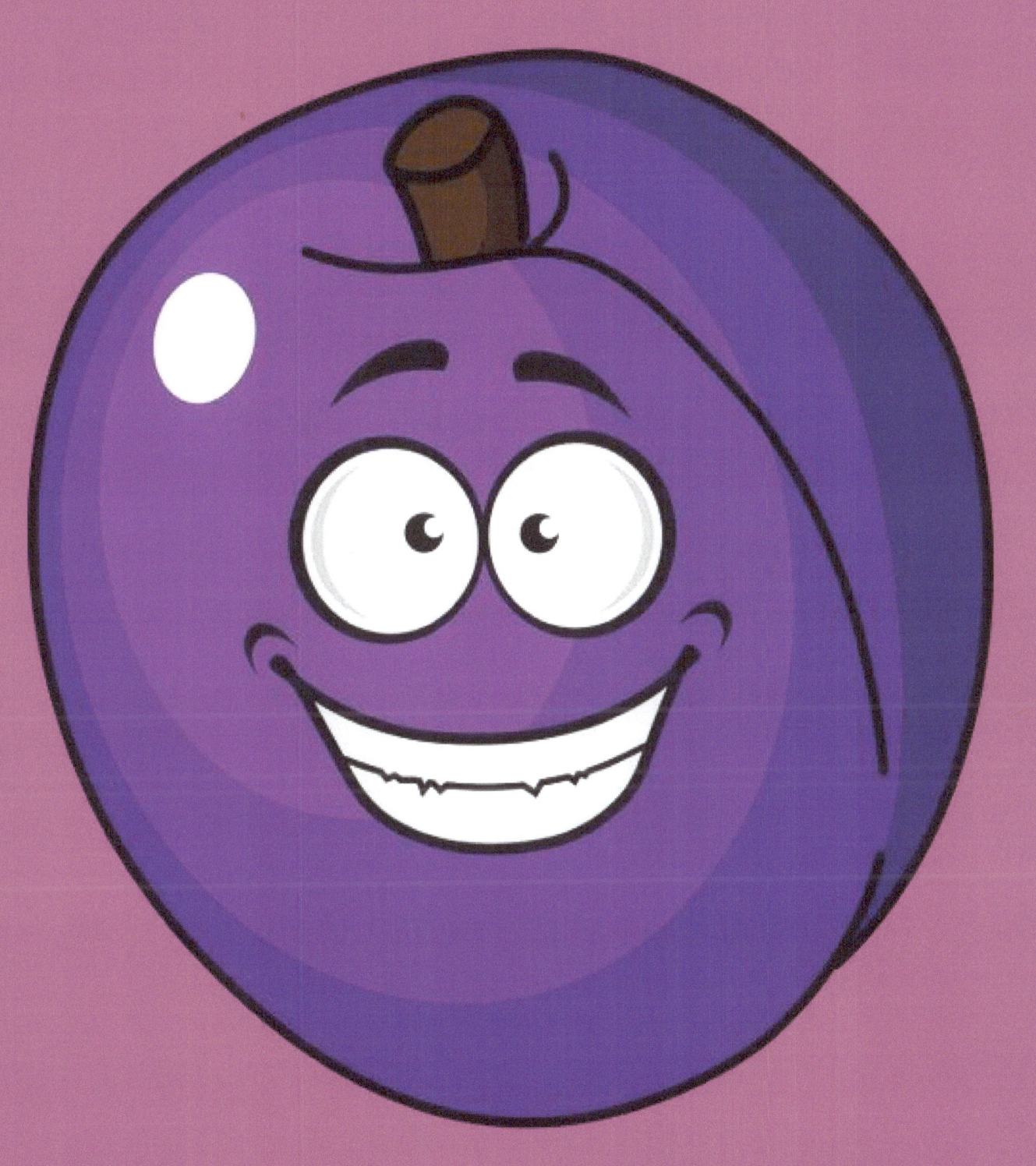

C c

is for Cherry

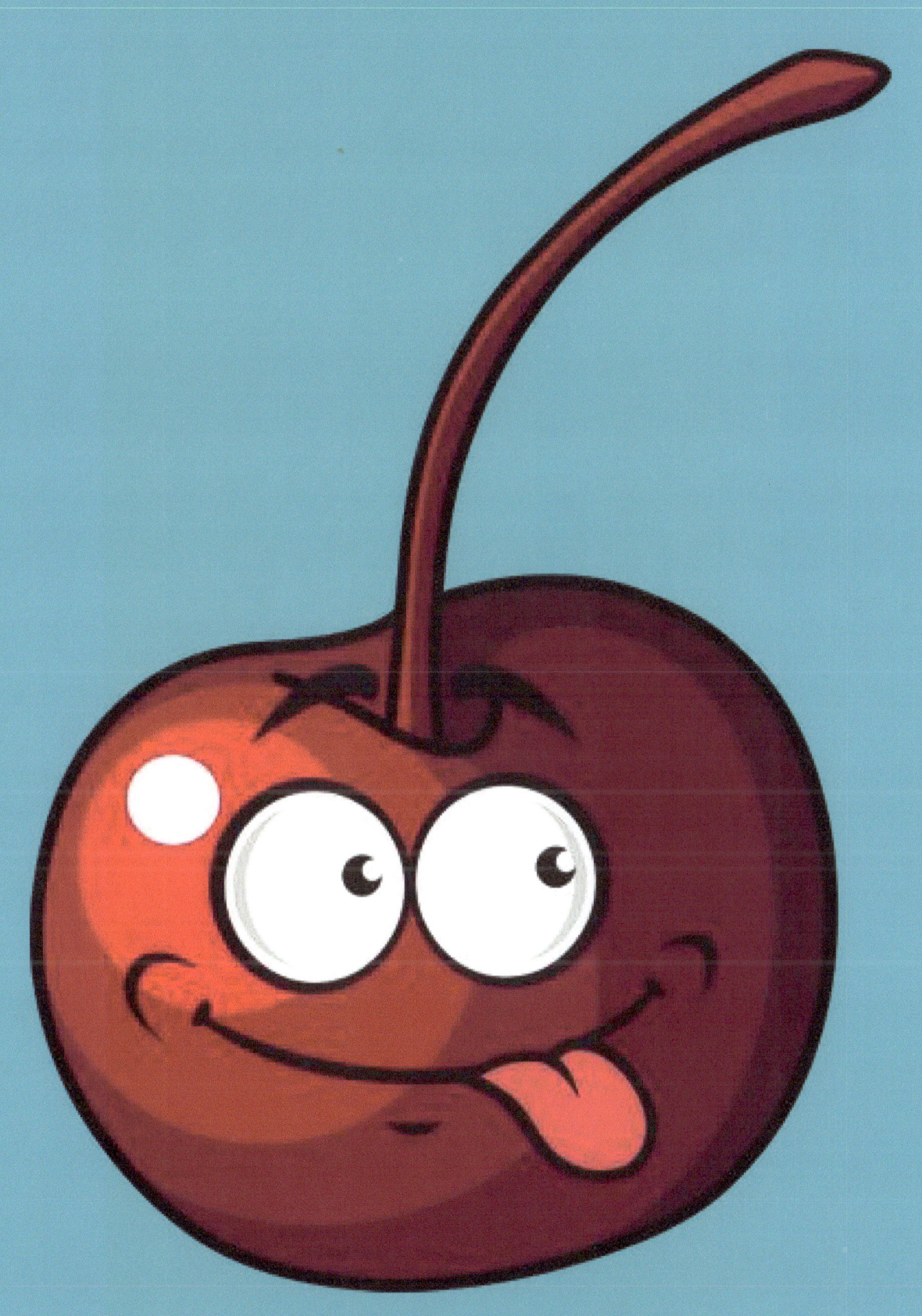

D d

is for Durian

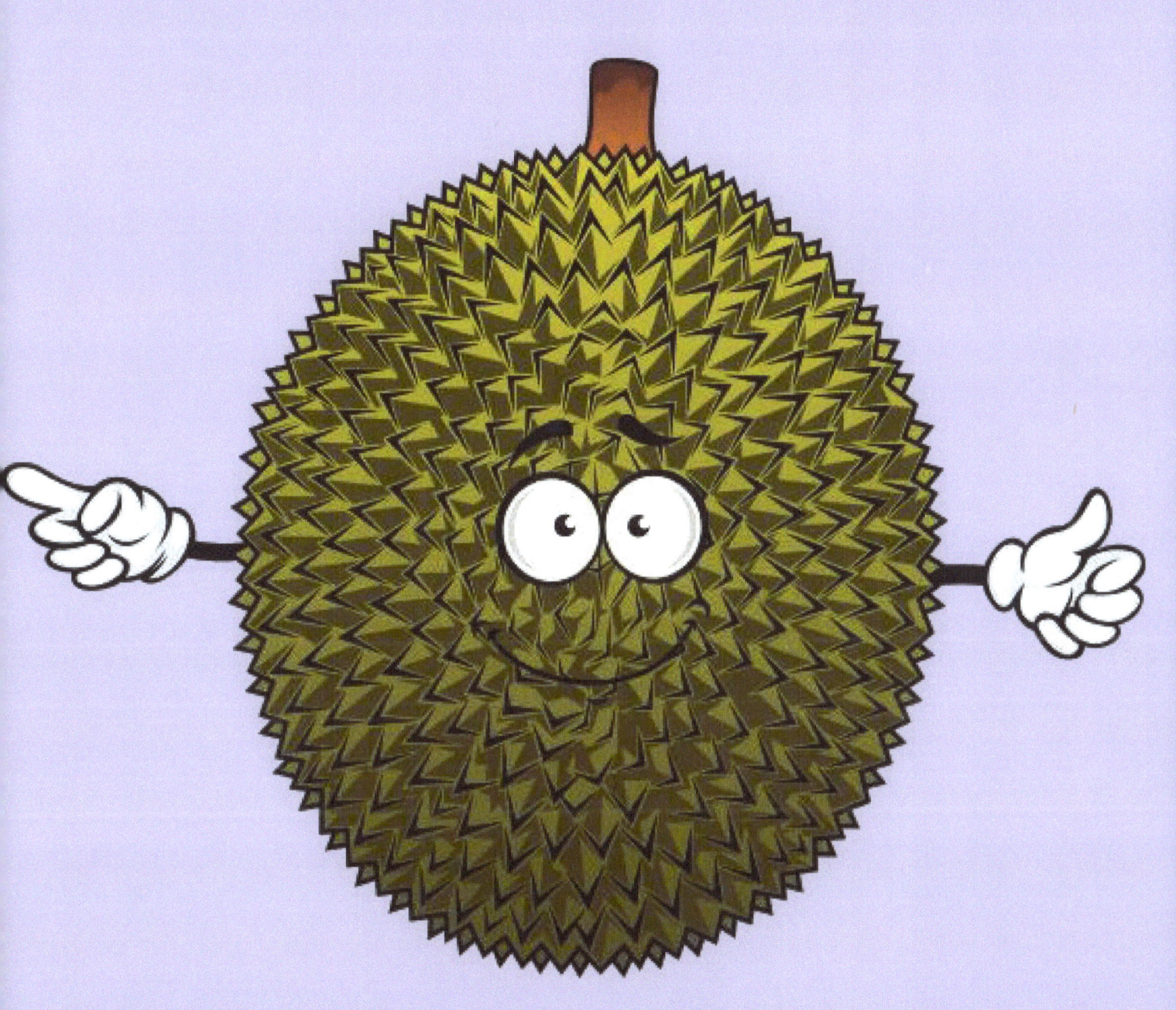

F f

is for Fig

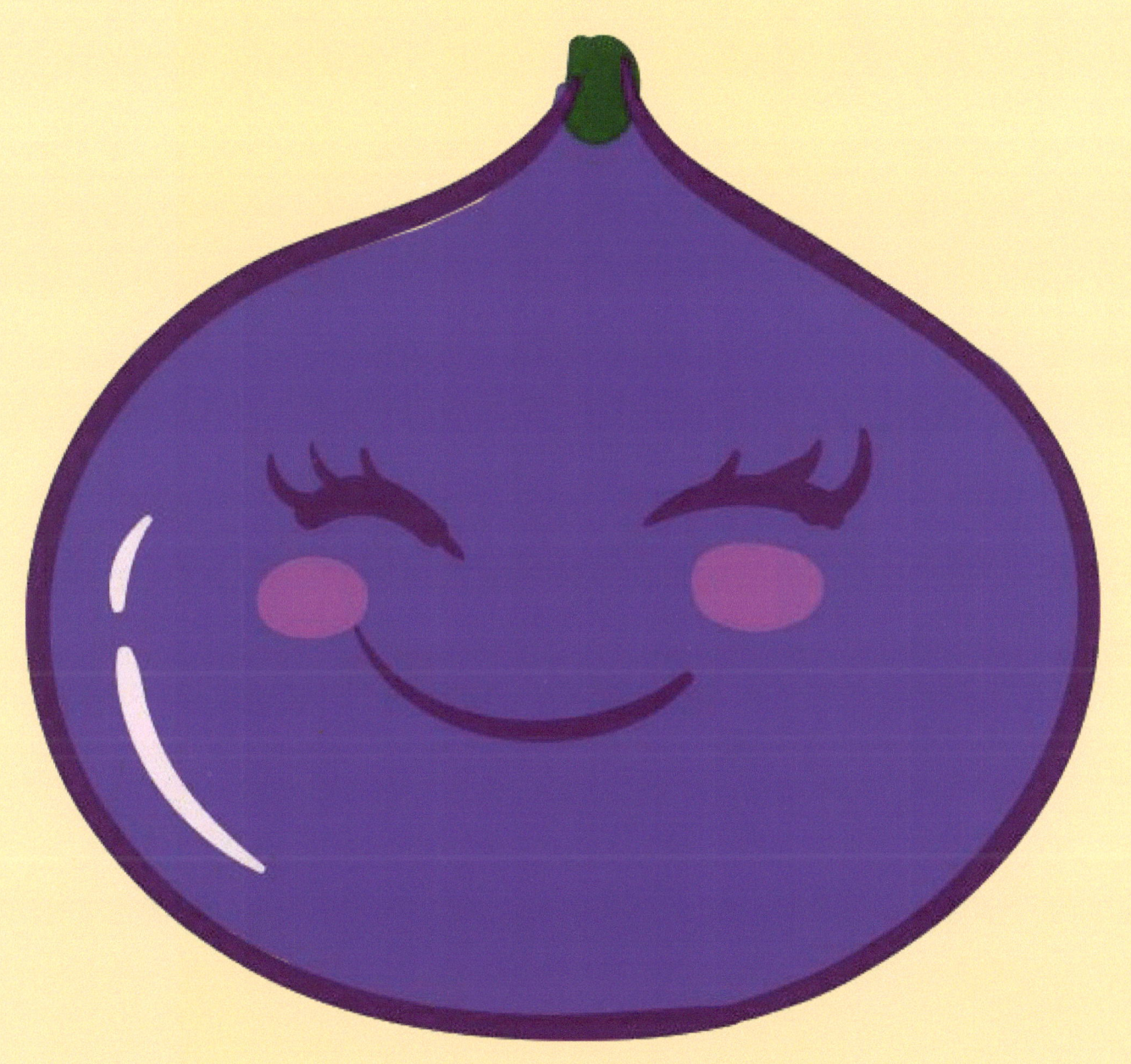

G g

is for Grapes

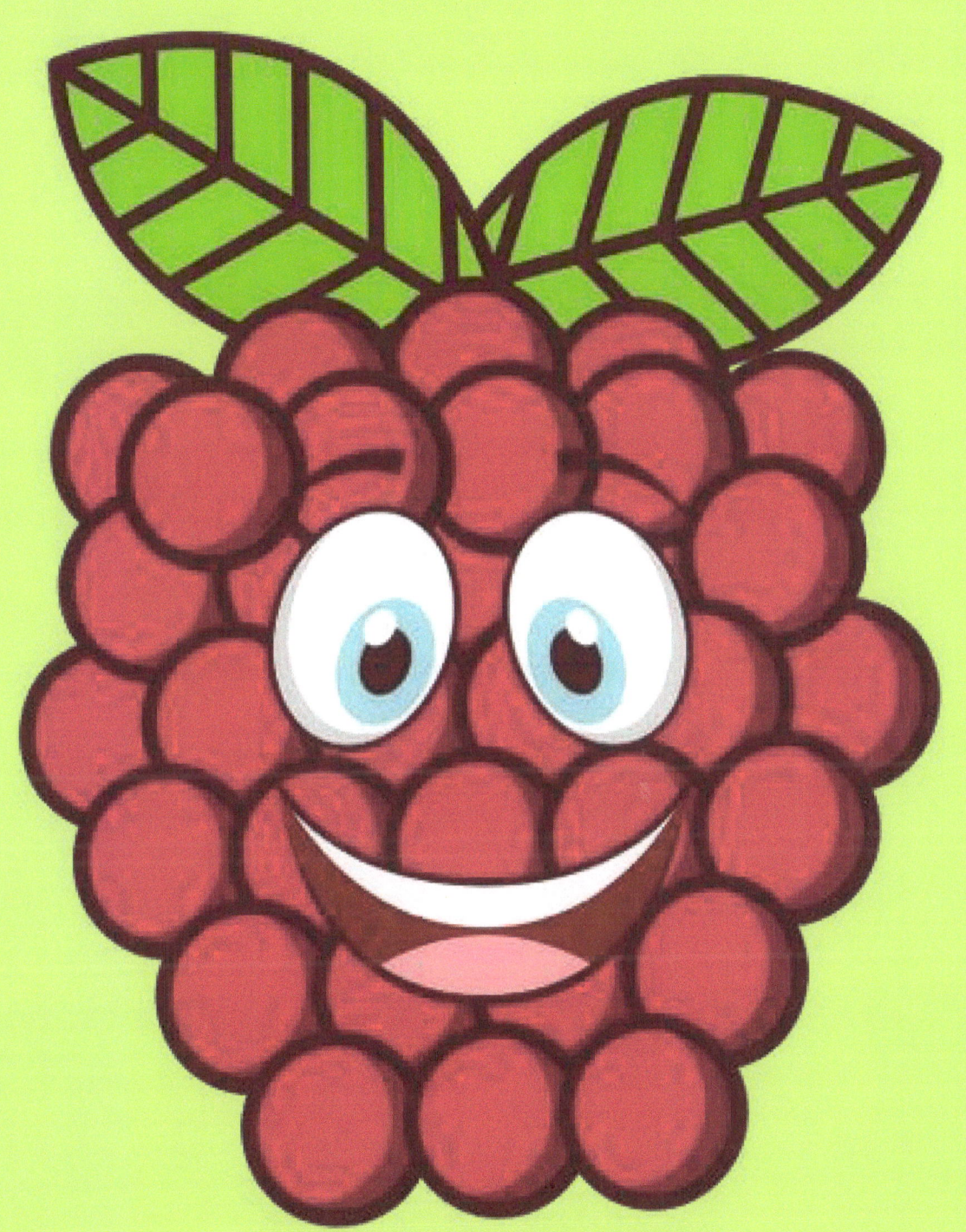

Jj

is for Jackfruit

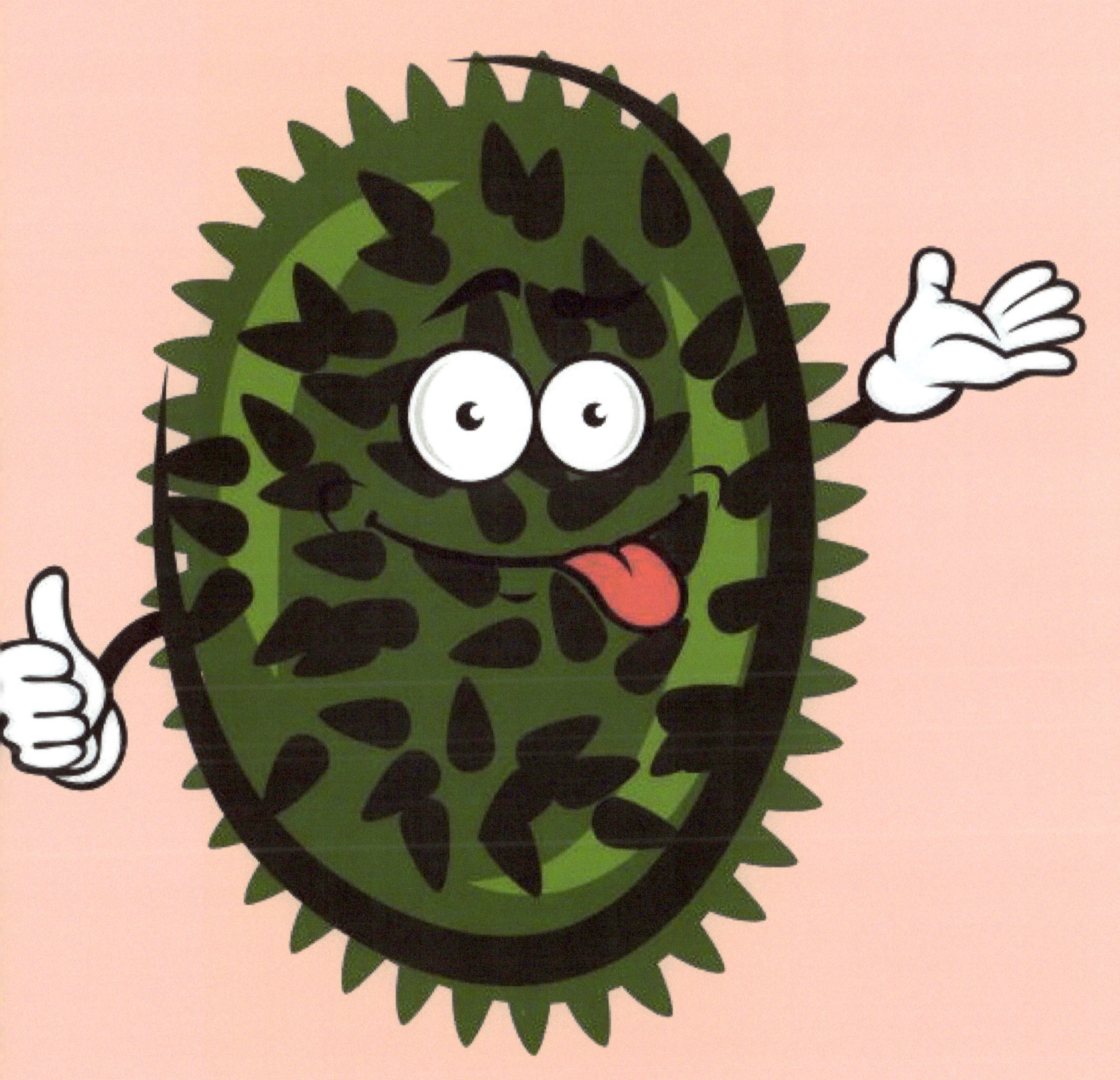

K k

is for Kiwi

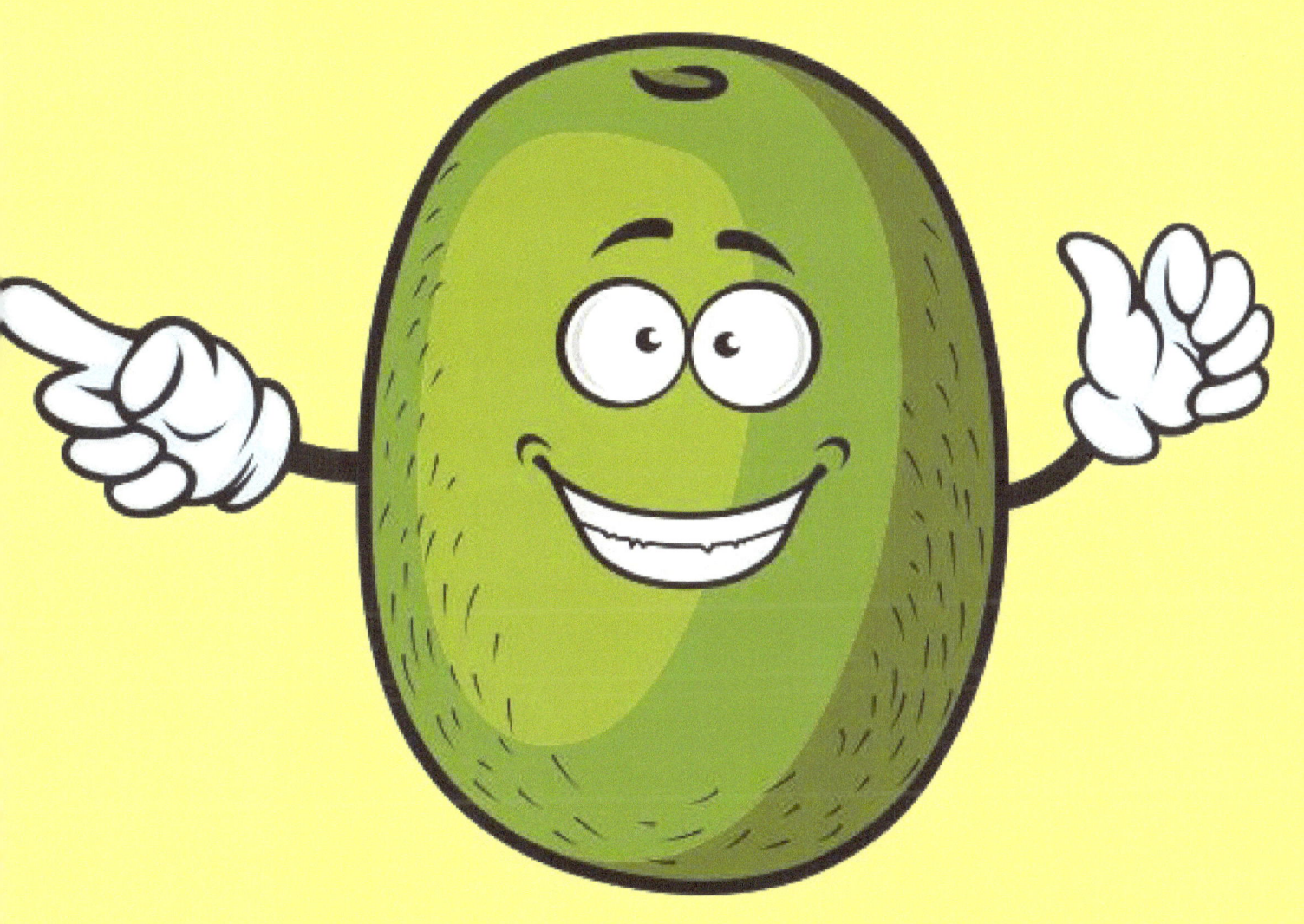

Ll

is for Lemon

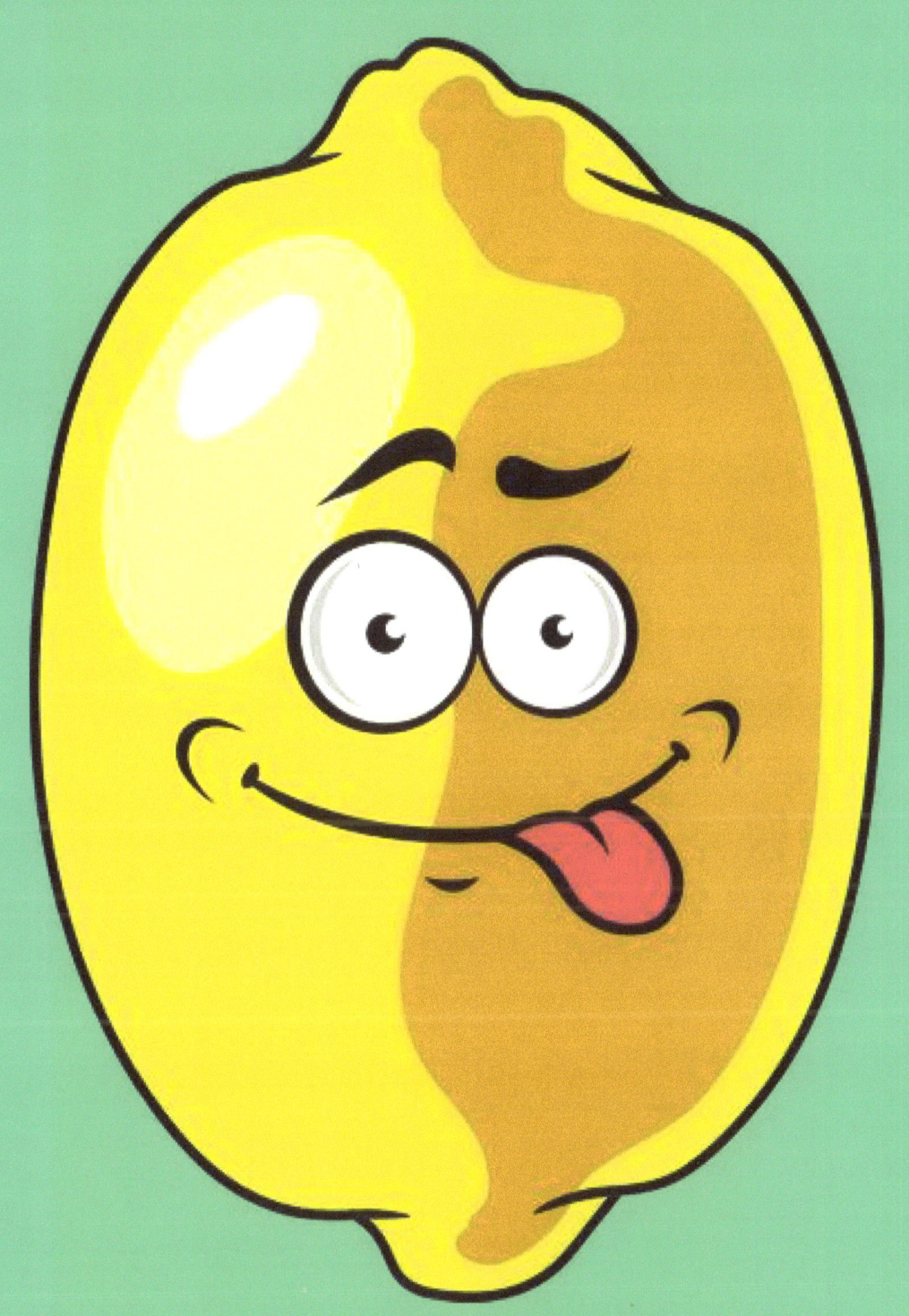

M m

is for Mango

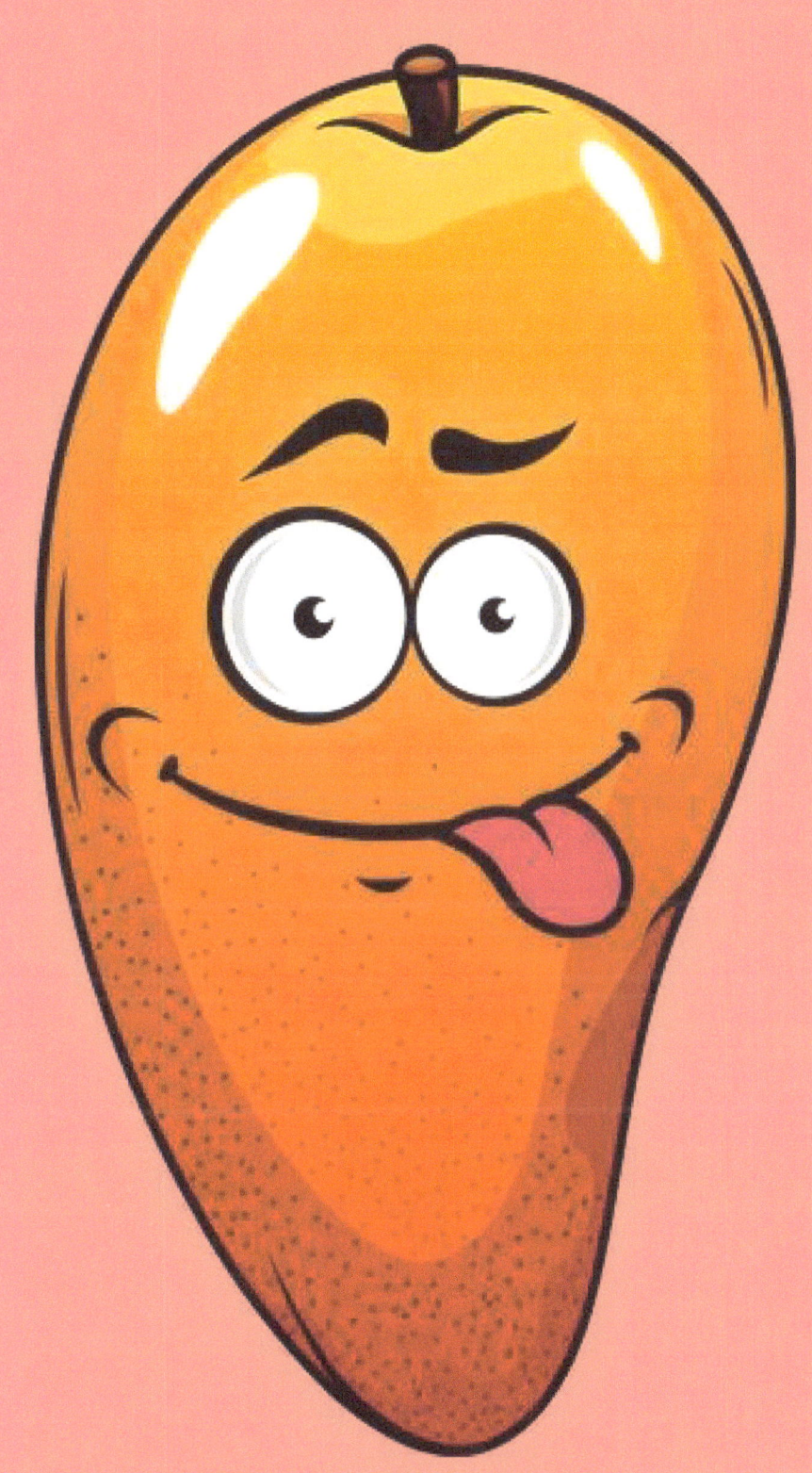

N n

is for Nectarine

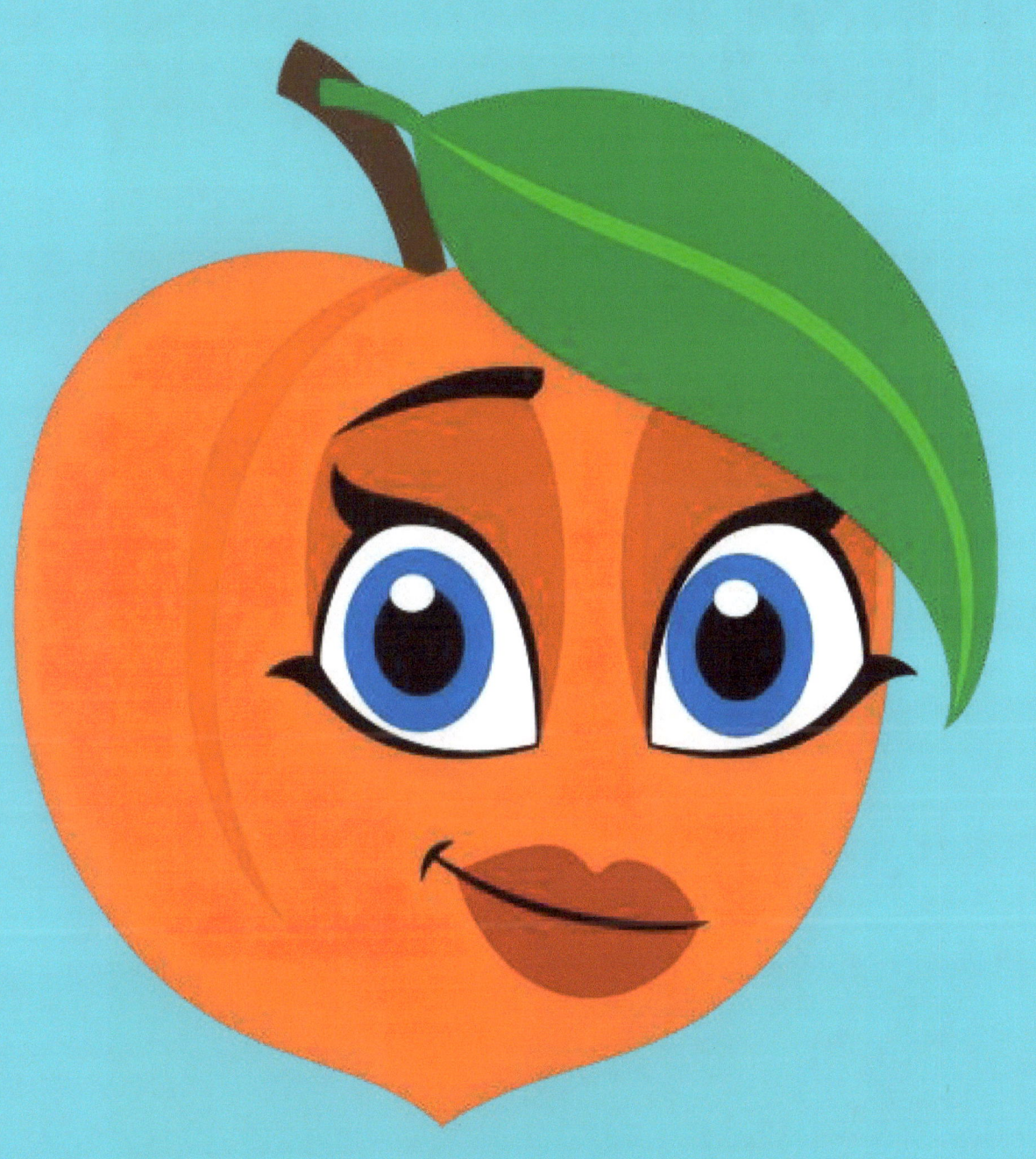

O o

is for Orange

P p

is for Pear

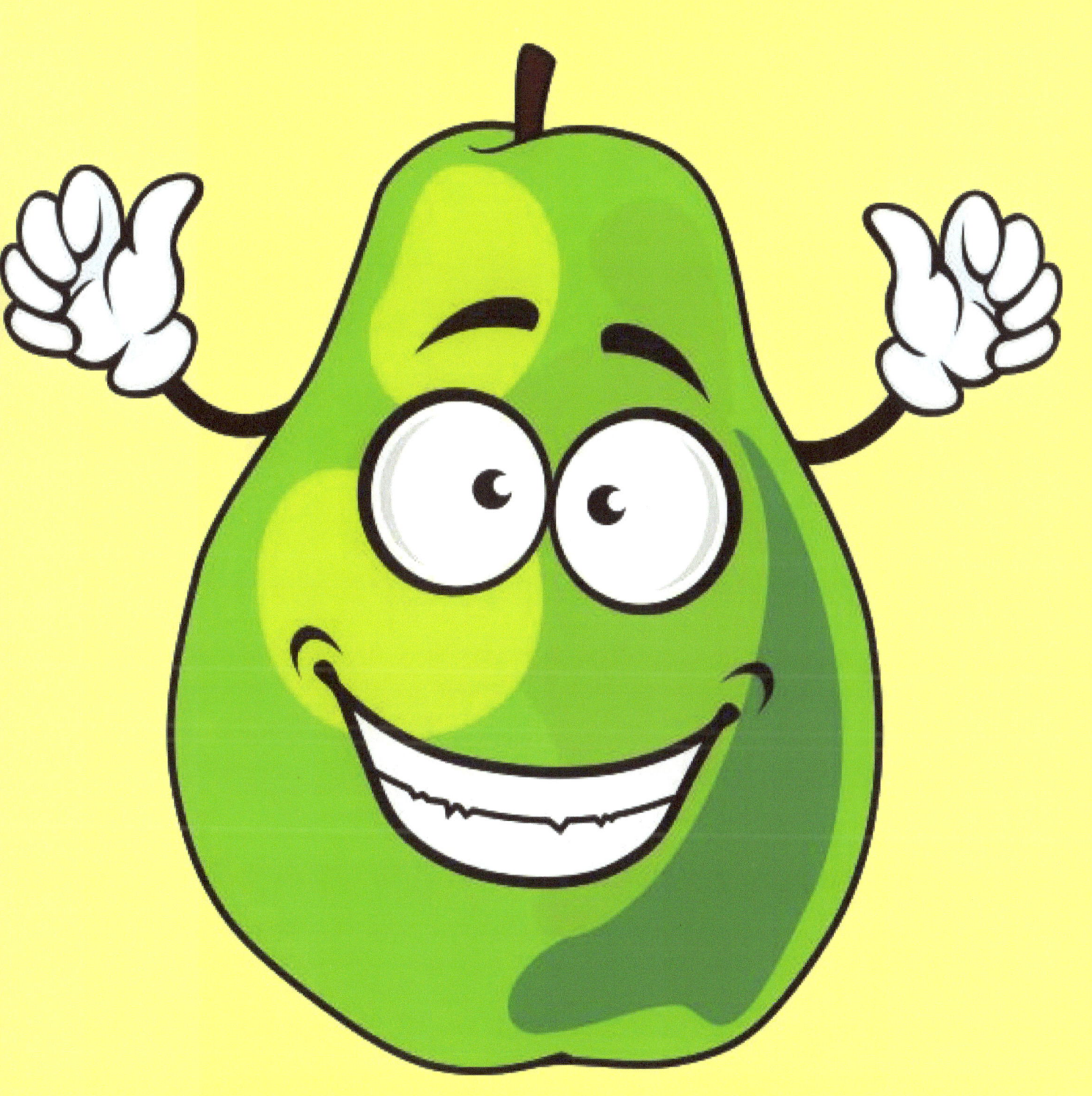

R r

is for Raspberry

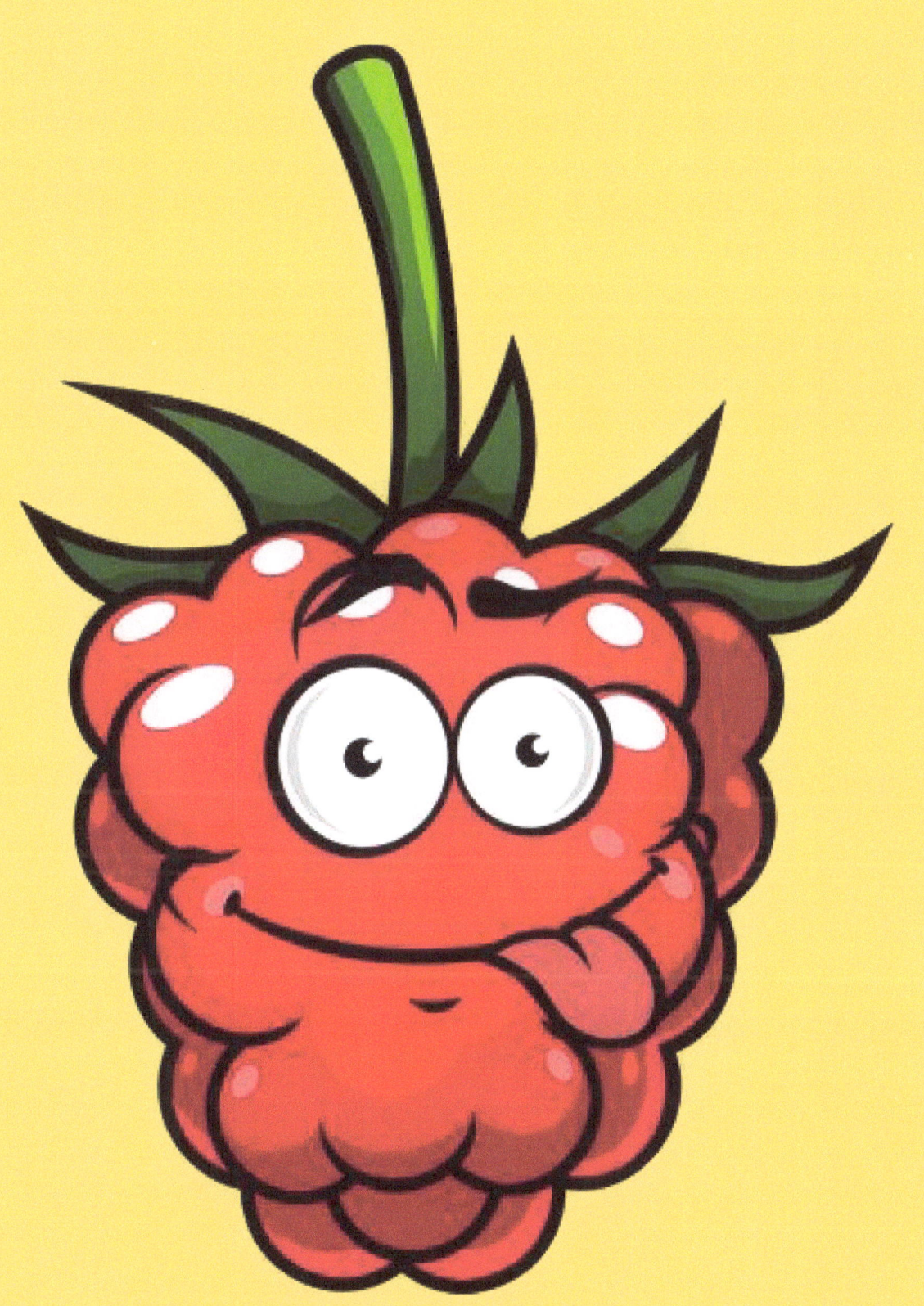

S s

is for Strawberry

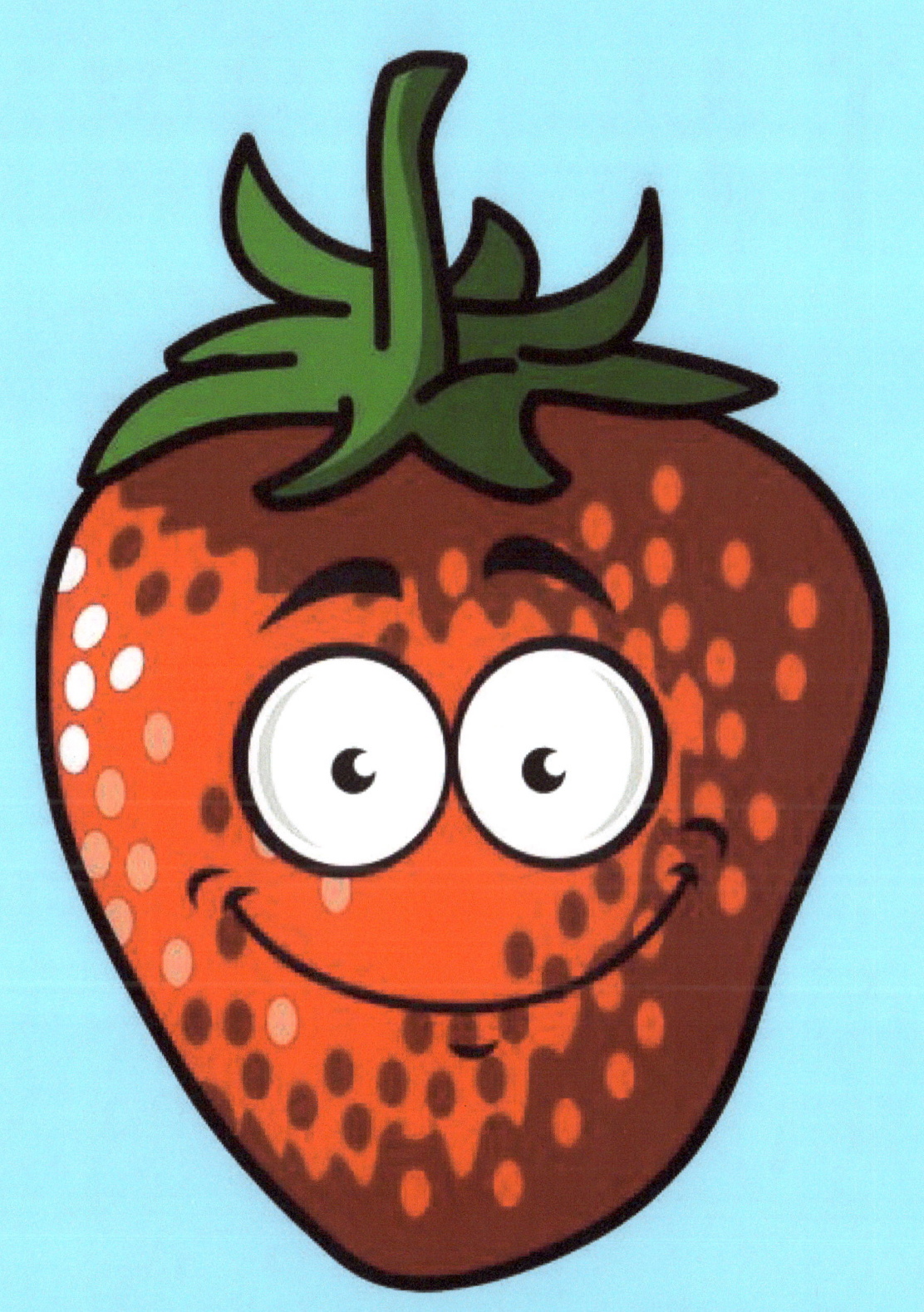

T t

is for Tangerine

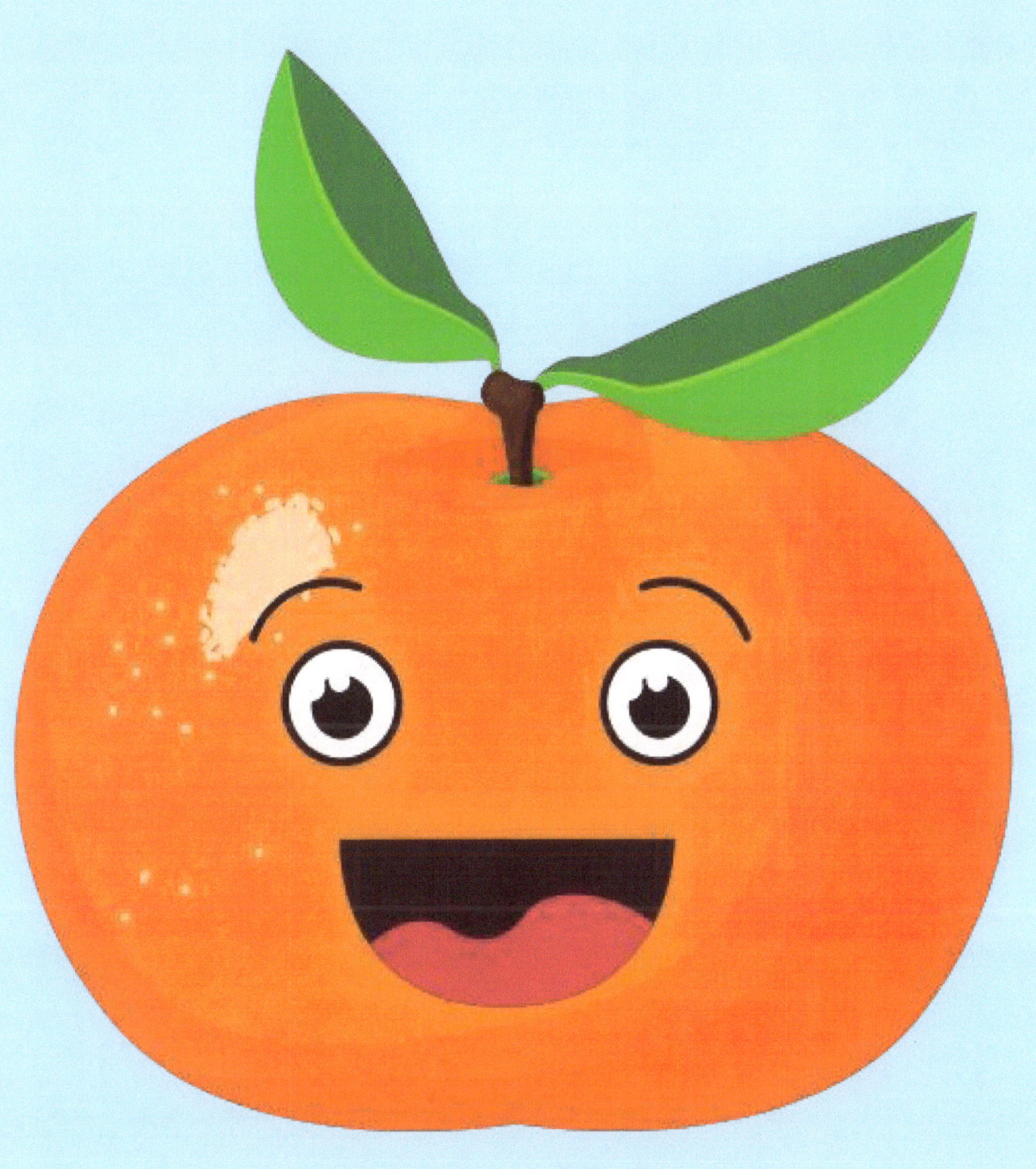

W w

is for Watermelon

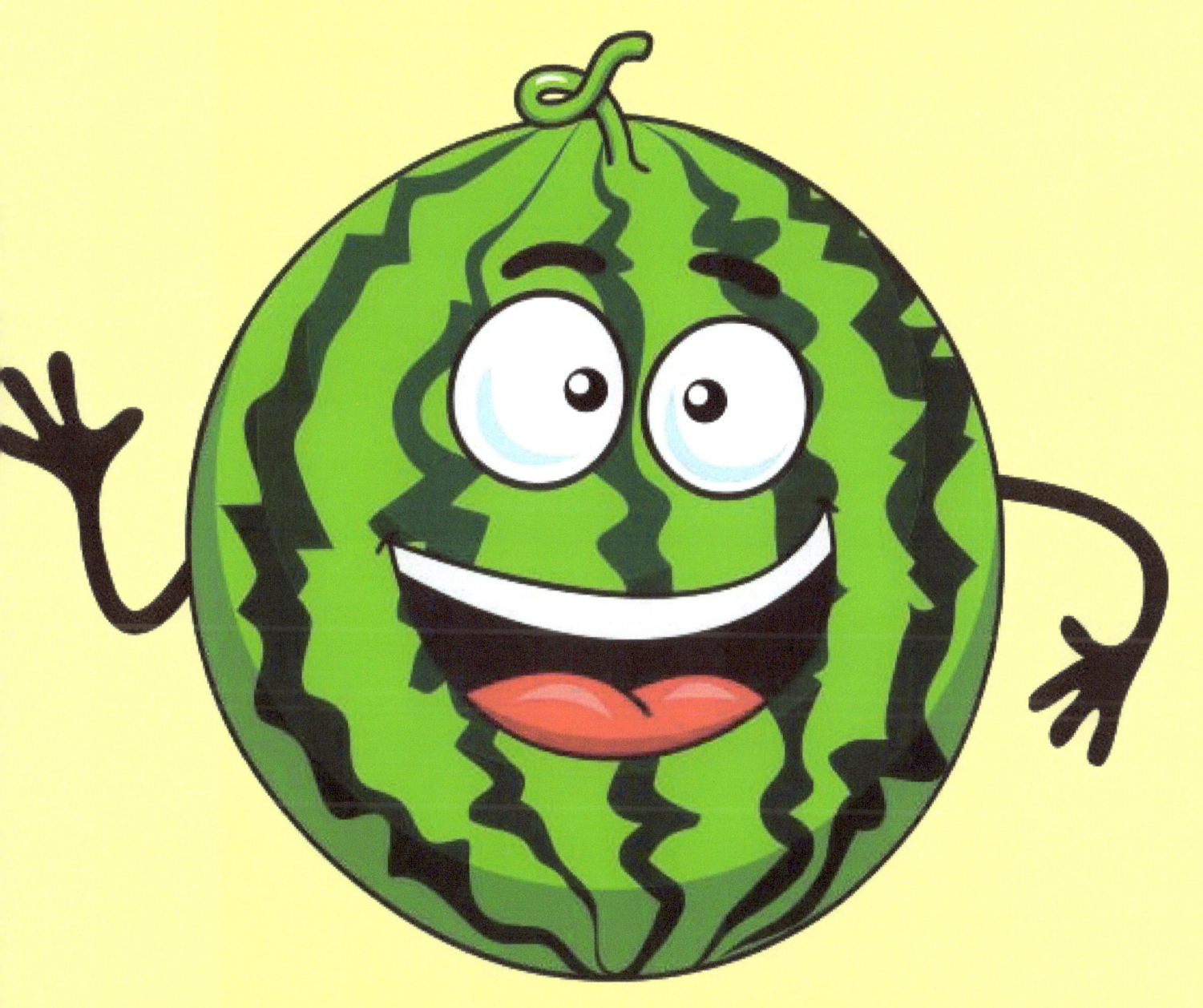

Zz

is for Zucchini

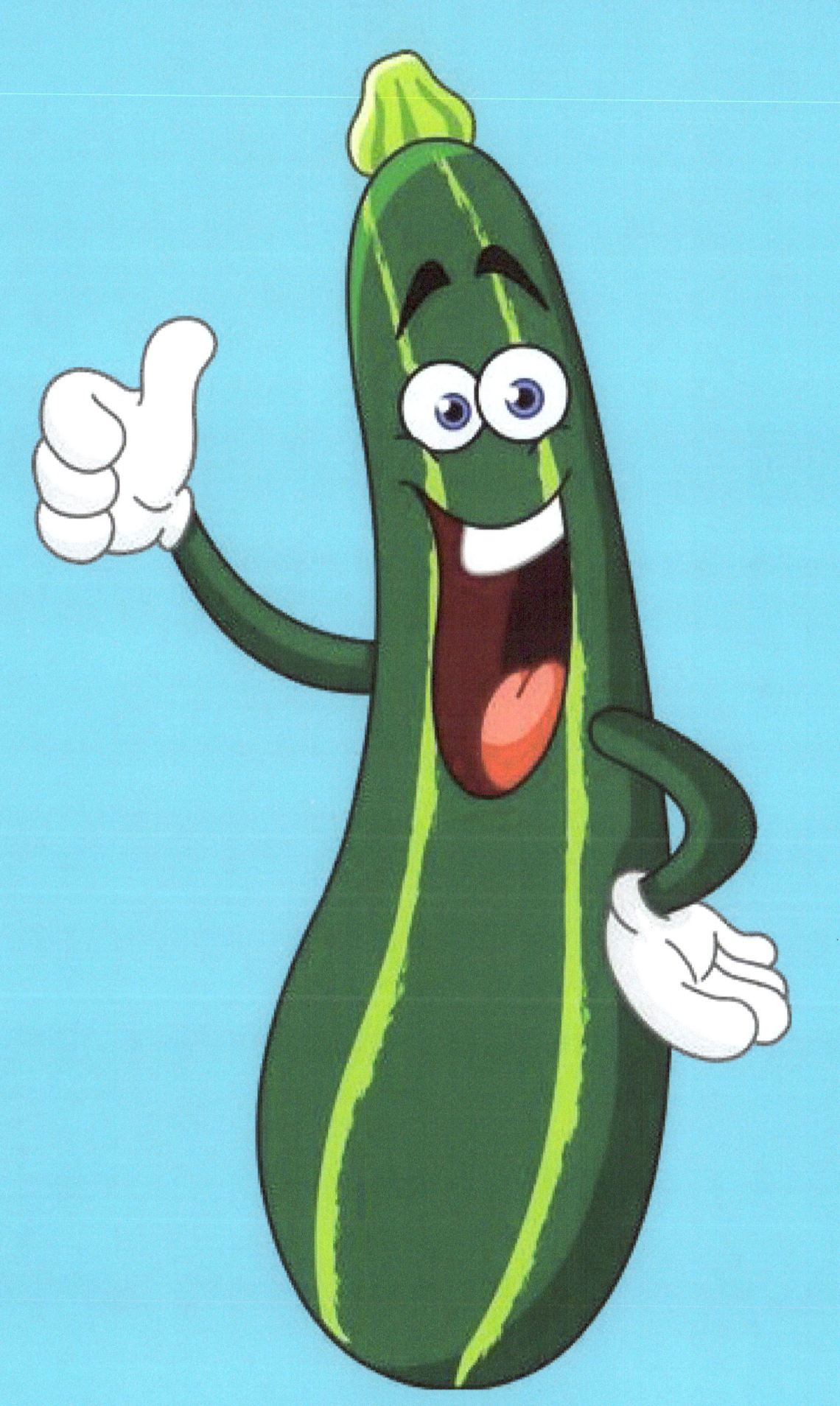